50+ Mediterranean Recipes Ideas

Need New Ideas for a Better Meal? Try These Tasty Recipes

Joseph Bellisario

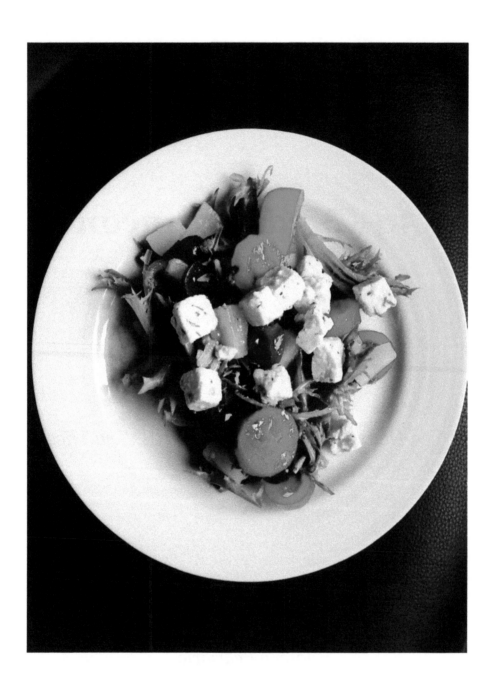

TABLE OF CONTENTS

Pressure pot mujadara

Ingredients

- ½ teaspoon of cinnamon
- 1 teaspoon of allspice
- 1 cup of brown lentils
- lemon zest from 1 small lemon
- 1 ½ tablespoons of olive oil
- 3 cups of water
- 3 fat shallots, thinly sliced
- 4 cloves garlic, rough chopped
- 2 teaspoons of cumin
- ¼ teaspoon of ground ginger
- 1 teaspoons of coriander
- 1 cup of brown basmati rice
- 1 teaspoon of dried mint
- ½ teaspoon of turmeric
- 1 ½ teaspoons of kosher salt

Directions

1. Place lentils in a bowl and cover with hot tap water.
2. Sauté shallots in olive oil for 5 minutes, stirring constantly.
3. Remove half , saving for the topping.

4. Add the garlic and sauté until fragrant.

5. Add all the spices, salt , lemon zest, and water. Stir.

6. Drain the lentils and add them with the rice to the Pressure pot. Stir.

7. Cover, set to high pressure for 11 minutes.

8. Let naturally release for 10 minutes.

9. Gently fluff the Mujadara with a fork.

10. Divide among bowls, drizzle with olive oil .

11. Add tomatoes, avocado together with the caramelized shallots, sprouts, a spoonful of yogurt.

12. Enjoy.

Grilled eggplant salad with freekeh and yogurt dressing

Ingredients

- 4 tablespoons of olive oil
- 1 cup of dry freekeh
- 2 ½ cups of water
- Sumac
- 2 garlic cloves finely minced
- ½ teaspoon of pepper
- 1 large eggplant, sliced
- Salt
- 1 cup of plain thick Greek yogurt
- ¼ cup of mint, chopped
- ½ teaspoon of Aleppo chili flakes
- 3 cup of dill, chopped
- ¼ cup Italian parsley, chopped
- 3 scallions, sliced
- 1 tablespoon of lemon zest
- 4 tablespoons of lemon juice

Directions

1. Preheat your grill to medium high.
2. Then, place freekeh with water in a medium pot.
3. Bring to a boil, cover, lower the heat, let simmer for 20 minutes.
4. Brush sliced eggplants with olive oil .
5. Season with salt, then, grill on both sides for 4 minutes.
6. Wrap in a foil, let steam and cook through. Cut into bite-sized pieces.
7. Combine cooked freekeh together with the eggplant, lemon zest, scallions, chopped herbs, olive oil , lemon juice, salt , pepper, and spices in a bowl. Toss.
8. Taste and adjust the seasoning with salt and lemon.
9. Combine yogurt, lemon juice, dill, garlic, sumac, and salt in a small bowl, whisk.
10. Serve and enjoy.

Grilled romaine salad with corn, fava beans, and avocado

Ingredients

- 1 tablespoon of lemon juice
- 2 romaine hearts
- 1 ear corn, shucked
- 6 tablespoons of olive oil
- 1 tablespoon of sherry vinegar
- 1 teaspoon of honey
- 1 teaspoon of sumac
- ¼ teaspoon of salt and pepper
- ½ pound fresh fava beans in pods
- 3 tablespoons of chopped dill
- 1 lemon
- ½ pound of shrimp
- 1 avocado, diced
- ½ teaspoon of salt
- 1-pint cherry tomatoes, cut in half.
- ½ cup plain yogurt
- 1 tablespoon lemon juice
- 2 fat clove garlic, finely minced

Directions

1. Preheat your grill to medium high.
2. Whisk together olive oil, sherry vinegar, lemon juice, honey, sumac, salt, and garlic, set aside.
3. Brush the romaine with olive oil.
4. Season with salt , then grill each side briefly until grill marks appear on. Keep on a platter.
5. Grill the lemon with the corn on the cob, fava beans, and shrimp over medium heat.
6. After 10 minutes, shuck and divide among the romaine wedges.
7. Cut the kernels off the corn and divide.
8. Add the diced avocado and halved cherry tomatoes.
9. Squeeze the salad with the grilled lemon halves, spoon a little dressing over top.
10. Scatter with fresh herbs.
11. Serve and enjoy.

Summer pasta salad with zucchini, corn, and cilantro pesto

Ingredients

- 6 ounces of rice noodles
- ½ teaspoon of smoked paprika
- ½ teaspoon of coriander
- ½ teaspoon salt
- 2 medium zucchini
- ¼ teaspoon of pepper
- 1 red bell pepper
- ½ of an onion
- 2 ears of fresh corn
- 1 tablespoon of lime zest
- ⅓ cup of pumpkin seeds
- Salt and pepper
- 1 large bunch cilantro and thin stems
- 2 fat garlic cloves
- 2 tablespoons of chopped jalapeno
- 2 tablespoons of lime juice
- ½ cup of olive oil

Directions

1. Preheat your grill ready to medium high.
2. Brush the veggie with olive oil and sprinkle with salt and pepper.
3. Pour boiling water over the rice noodles, drain and rinse. Keep aside.
4. Place the veggies on the grill, lower heat to medium, cover.
5. Place cilantro together with the garlic and jalapeño in a blender, pulse until finely chopped.
6. Add the remaining ingredients, pulse to combine. Not so smooth.
7. Cut the vegetables into bite-sized pieces, when they are done.
8. Loosen the pasta with cold water. Drain in dish.
9. Add the Cilantro Pesto with the veggies.
10. Taste, and a djust the seasoning accordingly.
11. Serve and enjoy topped with halved cherry tomatoes and lime wedges.

Lentil salad with spring veggies, mint, and yogurt sauce

Ingredients

- 2 garlic cloves finely minced
- 2 cups of cooked lentils
- 1 lemon, zest and juice
- 3 cups of spring veggies
- ¼ teaspoon of salt
- 2 tablespoons of fresh chopped dill
- Salt and pepper
- ½ teaspoon of sumac
- 3 tablespoons of red onion
- 2 garlic cloves
- ¼ cup of chopped mint leaves
- 2 tablespoons of olive oil
- 1 teaspoon of sumac
- 1 cup of plain thick Greek yogurt
- 1 tablespoon of lemon juice

Directions

1. Start by cooking the lentils in salted water until tender.
2. Slightly steam the veggies.

3. Place the lentils together with the veggies, onion, garlic, and mint in a bowl.
4. Toss with the olive oil , lemon zest, and lemon juice.
5. Season with salt , pepper, and sumac.
6. Mix Greek yogurt, lemon juice, dill, garlic, sumac, and salt in a small bowl
7. Smear the yogurt sauce on a platter topping with lentil salad.
8. Serve and enjoy.

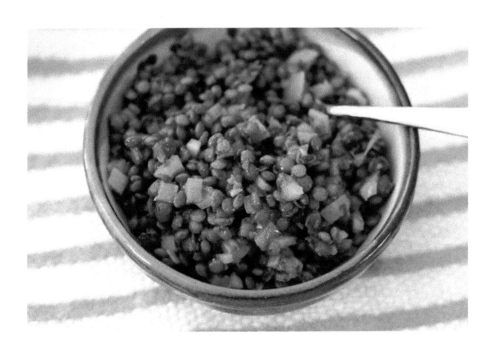

Creamy polenta with spring veggies and gremolata

Ingredients

- 1 cup of mushrooms
- ½ cup of dry polenta
- 2 cups asparagus
- 1 teaspoon of fresh thyme
- ¾ teaspoon of salt
- 1 teaspoon of granulated onion powder
- ¼ teaspoon of pepper
- 2 ½ cups of water
- 4 tablespoons of olive oil
- 2 tablespoons of gremolata
- 5 cups of veggies
- 1 shallot, chopped
- 1 cup of porcini mushrooms
- 1 cup of fiddlehead ferns
- Handful of pea shoots
- 2 tablespoons of sherry wine
- Salt and pepper

Directions

1. Bring water to boil in a medium pot .
2. Season with salt , pepper, and spices.
3. Gradually whisk in the dry polenta, let simmer for 10 minutes covered over low heat.
4. Continue to cook for another 10 minutes.
5. Stir in the olive oil. Switch off heat source.
6. In a large skillet, heat olive oil over medium heat.
7. Add mushrooms, let sauce until tender.
8. Add shallot and other veggies.
9. Season with salt and pepper, stir.
10. Lower heat, continue to cook for 5 minutes until fork tender.
11. Serve and enjoy.

Vegan green goddess bowl

Ingredients

- 1 tablespoon of vinegar
- 1 tablespoon of water
- 4 radishes, sliced
- 1 cucumber, sliced into ribbons
- 1 teaspoon of kosher salt
- 10 green beans
- 1 carrot, sliced into ribbons
- 1 tablespoon of lemon
- 3 tablespoons of olive oil
- 1 teaspoon of white miso paste
- 1 avocado, sliced in half
- 1 cup of shelled edamame
- 6 small potatoes
- 10 asparagus spears
- 1 package of silken tofu
- 2 fat garlic cloves
- 1 fat scallion, white and green parts
- 1 cup of fresh herbs
- ½ teaspoon of pepper

Directions

1. Bring salted water to a simmer on the stove.
2. Add the whole potatoes, cover and simmer until fork tender.
3. Remove the potatoes, set aside, keep warm.
4. Place in the edamame together with the asparagus, and green beans into the same hot water, continue to simmer briefly until tender and bright green. Strain.
5. Divide between two bowls and serve with dressing.
6. Place silken tofu, garlic, scallion, herbs, olive oil, lemon, vinegar, water, kosher salt, miso, and pepper in a blender.
7. Blend until smooth.
8. Taste and adjust seasoning.
9. Serve and enjoy.

Blackened tempeh with kale and avocado

Ingredients

- 1 scallion, sliced
- ⅓ cup of vegan ranch dressing
- Cajun spice blend
- Pinch salt, lemon zest from ½ a lemon
- ¼ cup of pickled onions
- 1 block tempeh
- 2 tablespoons of olive oil
- 1 avocado, sliced
- 5 leaves of lacinato kale
- 1 teaspoon of oil
- 4 radishes, sliced

Directions

1. Firstly, stir the spice into the dressing.
2. Taste, and adjust accordingly.
3. Add the tempeh, and sauté pan with salted water, enough to cover.
4. Let simmer for 10 minutes to reduce bitterness.
5. Slice and coat each side with Cajun Spices.

6. Then, pan-sear the tempeh in bit of oil, until crispy. Set aside.
7. Stack the kale, cut in to thin ribbons.
8. Place in a bowl and add a teaspoon, a pinch of salt and lemon zest.
9. Massage with your fingers until tender.
10. Add the radishes together with the scallion, pickled onion, and avocado to the kale.
11. Toss with some of the Vegan Ranch dressing to coat.
12. Divide the salad among bowls top with the blackened tempeh and sprouts.
13. Serve and enjoy.

Tarragon chicken with asparagus, lemon, and leeks

Ingredients

- 2 large leeks, sliced
- 1 extra-large bunch asparagus
- ½ teaspoon of pepper
- 2 lemons
- 2 teaspoons of salt
- 1/ 4 cup of olive oil
- 6 garlic cloves, finely minced
- 1-ounce package of fresh tarragon leaves
- 1.5 lbs. chicken breast

Directions

1. Place the zest of 1 lemon with its juice in a small bowl.
2. Then, add olive oil, garlic, salt and pepper, mix until salt dissolves.
3. Add ½ of the fresh tarragon, saving the balance for garnish.
4. Place the asparagus in a bowl and spoon some of the marinade over top.

5. Toss to combine, then place on a parchment lined sheet pan .
6. Add leeks to the same bowl, toss with a little marinade and spread out on the sheet pan .
7. Add the chicken breasts, with the remaining marinade, coat.
8. Nestle the chicken amongst the asparagus.
9. Zest the second lemon over the whole sheet-pan, slice the lemons into rounds, layering them over the asparagus.
10. Let bake for 20 minutes until golden.
11. Remove, toss to coat the chicken top with the flavorful juices.
12. Serve and enjoy.

Curry tofu salad

Ingredients

- 3 tablespoons of vegan mayo
- ½ teaspoon of cayenne pepper
- 8 ounces of tofu- extra firm
- 1 tablespoon of olive oil
- ¼ cup of cilantro, chopped
- 1 tablespoon of apple cider vinegar
- ¼ teaspoon of salt and pinch pepper
- ¼ cup of cashews, chopped
- ¼ cup of golden raisins
- ½ cup of celery, chopped
- Salt and pepper
- ¼ cup red onion, diced
- ½ cup of apple, diced
- 1 tablespoon of honey
- 3 teaspoons of curry powder

Directions

1. Begin by squeezing any excess water out of the tofu with a paper towel.
2. Then, cut into small cubes, blot again.
3. In a large skillet heat olive oil over medium heat.

4. Add salt and pepper to the olive oil then add tofu.
5. Sear on all sides until deeply golden, with a spatula turn, repeatedly.
6. Add raisins together with the onions, celery, cashews, apple, cilantro, stir.
7. Add spices, vegan mayo honey, and vinegar.
8. Season with salt and pepper.
9. Stuff into pitas with a handful of greens, or stuff avocados
10. Serve and enjoy.

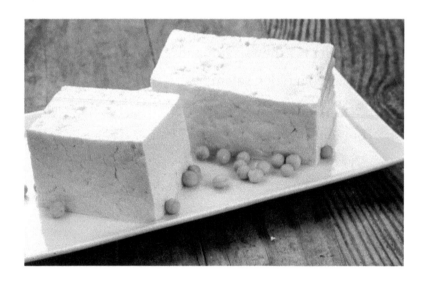

Beet noodles with yogurt and dill

Ingredients

- 1 tablespoon fresh dill, chopped
- 1 tablespoon of olive oil
- Salt and pepper to taste
- 1 fat shallot
- ¼ cup of water
- Toasted pine nuts
- 2 garlic cloves, rough chopped
- 6 ounces of beet noodles
- 3 tablespoons of plain yogurt

Direction

1. In a large skillet, heat the oil over medium heat.
2. Add the shallot together with the garlic and beet noodles, let sauté for 4 minutes, until golden and fragrant.
3. Add the water, let simmer for 6 minutes covered or until beet noodles are tender.
4. Uncover and continue to simmer.
5. Swirl in the yogurt and stir in the fresh dill.
6. Season with salt and pepper.
7. Top with toasted pine nuts and fresh dill.

8.   Serve and enjoy immediately.

Sweet and sour chicken

Ingredients

- Groundnut oil
- 100g of tender stem broccoli
- 1 x 227g tin of pineapple in natural juice
- 100g of baby sweetcorn
- 1 x 213g tin of peaches in natural juice
- 7cm piece of ginger
- ½ a bunch of fresh coriander
- 1 tablespoon of low-salt soy sauce
- 2 teaspoons of corn flour
- 1 yellow pepper
- 2 x 120g of chicken breasts
- Chinese five-spice
- 1 lime
- 2 cloves of garlic
- 1 bunch of asparagus
- 1 small onion
- 2 fresh red chilies
- 1 tablespoon of fish sauce
- 1 red pepper
- 1 teaspoon of runny honey

Directions

1. Drain the juices from the tinned fruit into a bowl.
2. To it, add the soy and fish sauces, whisk in half of corn flour until smooth.
3. Lay chicken skin in a large, cold frying pan, place on a low heat, briefly to render the fat, turning occasionally.
4. Remove once golden, add a pinch of sea salt and five-spice.
5. Place chunks of the chicken in a bowl together with 1 heaped teaspoon of five-spice, a pinch of salt, 1 teaspoon of corn flour, garlic, and half the lime juice.
6. Place a frying pan on a high heat, cook the chicken for 6 minutes, turning halfway, leave on a low heat.
7. Place a work on a high heat, scatter in the pepper and onion to scald and char for 5 minutes.
8. Add 1 tablespoon of olive oil, ginger, garlic, chilies, peaches, pineapple, baby sweetcorn, asparagus, and broccoli.
9. Stir-fry for 3 minutes, pour in the sauce, cook briefly loosening splash of boiling water.
10. Drizzle the honey into the chicken pan, raise the heat to high, toss until sticky.
11. Serve and enjoy with the coriander leaves and lime wedges for squeezed.

Peanut butter oatmeal cookies

This is a gluten free recipe deliciously worth making at home at your time.

Ingredients

- 2 teaspoons of vanilla extract
- 2 ½ cups of packed coconut sugar
- Sea salt
- ⅓ cup of melted coconut oil
- 3 large eggs
- 1 ½ cups of creamy or chunky peanut butter
- 2 teaspoons of baking soda
- 2 ½ cups of quick-cooking oats

Directions

1. Preheat the oven to 350°F.
2. Then, align 2 baking sheets with parchment paper.
3. Combine the peanut butter together with the sugar and coconut oil in a mixing dish.
4. Mix until well combined in an electric mixer.
5. Add the eggs together with the baking soda and vanilla, mix well.

6. Add the oats mix to incorporate.

7. Place 2 tablespoons of dough per cookie onto the prepared baking sheets.

8. Shape the cookies into rounded mound and press down lightly.

9. Then, let bake for 10 minutes. Allow to cool for 10 minutes.

10. Transfer to a cooling rack.

11. Sprinkle with flaky sea salt.

12. Serve and enjoy.

Chocolate peanut butter crispy bars

The chocolate peanut butter bars are sweetened with natural sweeteners mainly honey, baked with wholesome pantry ingredients perfect for a Mediterranean diet breakfast.

Ingredients

- ½ cup of honey
- 1 ¼ cups of whole pecans
- ½ teaspoon of flaky sea salt
- ¾ cup of creamy peanut butter
- 1 ½ cups of chocolate chips
- 3 cups of brown rice crisps

Directions

1. Align a square baking dish with a strip of parchment paper
2. In a large mixing bowl, combine the brown rice crisps together with 1 cup of chopped pecans. keep for later.
3. In another saucepan, combine the peanut butter together with the honey.

4. Warm the mixture over medium-low heat, stirring often, until steaming in 5 minutes.

5. Pour the warm mixture into the bowl of rice crisps.

6. Stir until the mixture is completely combined.

7. Then, transfer to the lined baking dish.

8. Melt the chocolate chips for 30 seconds, stirring after each one.

9. Pour it over the peanut butter-crispy mixture. Spread with spatula evenly.

10. Sprinkle the remaining pecans on top, then with salt.

11. Refrigerate for at least 2 hours or more.

12. Slice, serve and enjoy.

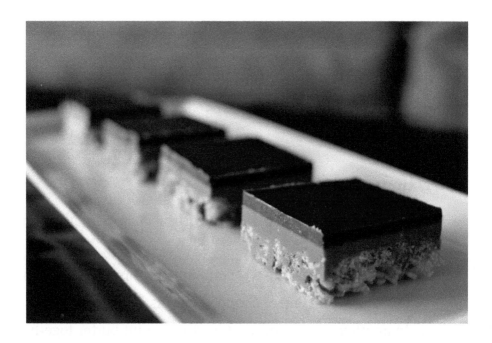

Healthier ginger bread cookies

Mediterranean Sea diet is a healthy choice of diet.

As a result, these ginger bread cookies have all the healthy properties for a perfect Mediterranean Sea diet.

Ingredients

- ¼ teaspoon of lemon zest
- 2 teaspoons of ground cinnamon
- ¾ teaspoon of kosher salt
- ½ teaspoon of finely ground black pepper
- 2 ¼ teaspoons of lemon juice
- ½ teaspoon of baking soda
- ½ cup of powdered sugar
- ¼ teaspoon of baking powder
- ½ cup melted coconut oil
- 3 cups of whole wheat pastry flour
- ½ cup of unsulphured molasses
- ½ cup of packed coconut sugar
- 1 large egg
- Powdered sugar
- ½ teaspoon of ground cloves
- 2 teaspoons of ground ginger

Directions

1. Combine the flour together with the ginger, salt, cloves, cinnamon, pepper, baking soda, and baking powder. Whisk to blended.
2. Then, combine the coconut oil with molasses, whisk to combined.
3. Add the coconut sugar, whisk.
4. Add the egg and whisk until the mixture is thoroughly blended.
5. Pour the liquid mixture into the dry, mix until combined.
6. Divide the dough in half. Shape each half into a round disc about, wrap in plastic wrap.
7. Refrigerate overnight.
8. Preheat your oven to 350°F.
9. Align 2 baking sheets with parchment paper.
10. Roll out one of the discs out until ¼ thick.
11. Place each cookie on a parchment-lined baking sheet.
12. Bake for 11 minutes, let cool.
13. Combine the powdered sugar with lemon zest and the lemon juice. Whisk to blend. Squeeze icing onto the cookies, let harden.
14. Serve and enjoy.

Peanut butter, banana, honey, and oat chocolate chip cookies

The ingredients of this Mediterranean diet recipe yield the highest health benefits especially the banana and oats.

It is a whole meal yet perfect foe breakfast and a snack.

Ingredients

- ½ teaspoon of baking powder
- ½ cup of natural unsalted peanut butter
- 4 tablespoons of unsalted butter, melted
- 1 large egg
- ½ teaspoon of baking soda
- ½ teaspoon of ground cinnamon
- ½ cup of honey or real maple syrup
- ⅓ cup of mashed overripe banana
- Flaky sea salt
- 1 ½ cups of old-fashioned rolled oats, ground
- 1 ½ cups of old-fashioned rolled oats
- ¾ teaspoon of fine-grain sea salt
- 1 ½ cups of semi-sweet chocolate chips
- 1 teaspoon of vanilla extract

Directions

1. Preheat your oven to 325°F.
2. Align 2 baking sheets with parchment paper.
3. Add honey to the ½ cup of lime with peanut butter until 1 cup total liquid line.
4. Pour the honey and peanut butter mixture into a mixing bowl.
5. Add the mashed banana together with the melted butter, whisk until to blend.
6. Beat in the egg, then whisk in the vanilla together with the baking soda, baking powder, salt, and cinnamon.
7. Stir in the ground oats with rolled oats, chocolate chips, and sprinkles until they are evenly combined.
8. Drop the dough by the heaping tablespoon onto prepared baking sheets.
9. Let bake while reversing the pans midway through until barely set within 16 minutes.
10. Remove, let them cool completely on the pans.
11. Serve and enjoy sprinkled with flaky salt.

Crispy baked tostones

The tostones uses green plantains as the main Mediterranean recipe ingredients with a delicious savory and salt to elevate its taste.

Ingredients

- Flaky sea salt
- 3 large unripe plantains
- 4 tablespoons avocado oil

Directions

1. Start by preheating your oven to 425°F.
2. Line a large baking sheet with parchment paper.
3. Toss the sliced plantains with 2 tablespoons of the oil in the baking sheet.
4. Disperse evenly across the pan.
5. Let bake for 15 minutes, then place the pan on a heat-safe surface.
6. Brush the tops of each round with oil, flip them and brush the other sides
7. Sprinkle with the salt.

8. Return the pan to the oven, let bake for 17 minutes, until golden.
9. Season with additional salt, to taste.
10. Serve and enjoy with dipping sauce.

Pecan sweet potato casserole

Ingredients

- ½ stick of unsalted butter, melted
- ¼ cup of packed coconut sugar
- Pinch of fine salt
- ½ cup of milk of choice
- ¾ cup of pecan halves
- ¼ cup of maple syrup
- ½ teaspoon of vanilla extract
- 3 pounds of sweet potatoes
- 2 teaspoons of finely snipped fresh rosemary leaves
- ½ teaspoon of ground cinnamon
- ¼ teaspoon of ground nutmeg
- ½ teaspoon of fine salt
- 3 tablespoons of unsalted butter

Directions

1. Preheat the oven to 425°F.
2. Line a baking sheet with parchment paper.
3. Grease a square baker with butter.
4. Prick sweet potatoes with a fork about 5 times.
5. Place the whole sweet potatoes on the prepared baking sheet, let bake for 45 minutes to 1 hour.

6. Lower the heat to 350°F. Scoop the insides of potatoes into a large mixing bowl.

7. Add the melted butter together with the maple syrup, vanilla, milk, nutmeg, and salt to the bowl.

8. Mix until smooth and creamy.

9. Scoop the mixture into the prepared baker and spread in an even layer.

10. In a medium bowl, combine the softened butter together with the, sugar, pecans, rosemary, cinnamon, and salt.

11. Stir until the mixture is evenly incorporated.

12. Let bake for 30 minutes, until the pecans are golden and fragrant.

13. Serve and enjoy.

Vegetarian succotash

This is a lovely gift for the Mediterranean Sea diet vegetarian lovers.

Packed with variety of vegetables typically pecans, basil, onions, and garlic among others for a greater flavor.

Ingredients

- Pinch of cayenne
- 2 tablespoons of extra virgin olive oil
- 1 teaspoon of fine salt, divided
- Flaky sea salt
- 1 small red onion, chopped
- ¼ cup of chopped fresh basil, divided
- 1 poblano pepper, chopped
- 2 tablespoons of chopped green onion
- 1 red bell pepper, chopped
- 2 cloves garlic, pressed
- 2 cups of fresh beans
- 4 ears of fresh corn, shucked
- 2 tablespoons of butter
- Freshly ground black pepper

Directions

1. Warm olive oil over medium-high heat, until starting to shimmer.
2. Add the corn with ½ teaspoon of the salt.
3. Let cook for 7 minutes, stirring frequently, until the corn is turning golden.
4. Lower the heat, then add the onion together with the poblano, bell pepper, jalapeño, and the remaining salt.
5. Stir to combine, cook, stirring often, until the onion is tender and turning translucent.
6. Add the garlic, stir to combine, let cook until fragrant.
7. Then, add the lima beans let cook for 2 minutes.
8. Add the butter to the skillet and stir until it's mostly melted.
9. Remove from the heat. Let cool briefly.
10. Taste, and adjust the seasoning.
11. Stir in about half of the basil, reserving some.
12. Transfer the succotash to a serving plate.
13. Serve and enjoy.

Mexican street corn

This corn is no ordinary corn, it is accompanied with chili powder, lime and mayonnaise for a better taste to suit the Mediterranean Sea diet taste.

It works as a snack or an appetizer.

Ingredients

- ¼ teaspoon of kosher salt
- 2 ounces of finely grated Cotjia cheese
- ¼ cup of mayonnaise
- 2 tablespoons of finely chopped cilantro
- 1 ½ teaspoons of lime juice
- ½ teaspoon of chili powder
- Pinch of cayenne pepper
- 4 ears of grilled corn on the cob

Directions

1. In a small bowl, combine the mayonnaise together with the lime juice, chili powder, cayenne, and salt. Stir to combined.
2. In another separate bowl, mix together the cheese with the cilantro. Set both aside for later.

3. Brush the mayonnaise mixture all over one ear of corn.

4. Sprinkle the Cotjia mixture liberally all over, turning the corn as needed.

5. Place the finished cob on a separate serving plate.

6. Repeat this step for the remaining corn.

7. Sprinkle a pinch of additional chili powder lightly over the corn.

8. Serve and enjoy when still warm.

Best guacamole

Ingredients

- 3 tablespoons of lime juice
- ¼ cup of finely chopped fresh cilantro
- 1 teaspoon of kosher salt
- 1 small jalapeño, seeds and ribs removed
- ½ cup of finely chopped white onion
- 4 medium ripe avocados
- ¼ teaspoon of ground coriander

Directions

1. Scoop the flesh of the avocados into a serving bowl.
2. Then, mash up the avocado until smooth to your expectation.
3. Next, add the onion together with the cilantro, coriander, jalapeño, lime juice, and salt. Stir until combine.
4. Taste, and adjust the seasoning to your taste.
5. Serve and enjoy.

Avocado pesto toast

Avocado is one of the few Mediterranean fruits blessed with the gift of nourishing the skin.

As a result, this recipe featuring tomatoes and garlic for a flavor is adequate for your skin nourishment needs.

Ingredients

- Cooked eggs
- 2 large ripe avocados
- Freshly ground black pepper, red pepper flakes
- 2 medium cloves garlic
- 2 tablespoons of lemon juice
- Halved cherry tomatoes
- ¼ teaspoon of salt
- ¼ cup of pepitas
- ⅔ cup of packed fresh basil leaves
- 4 slices of organic bread

Directions

1. Place the pepitas into a small skillet.
2. Let cook over medium heat, stirring frequently until making little popping noises.

3. Then, transfer to a bowl, let cool.
4. Scoop avocado flesh into a bowl of a food processor.
5. Place the garlic together with the lemon juice, and salt.
6. Blend until smooth.
7. Add the toasted pepitas with the basil leaves and pulse until the pepitas and basil are broken down.
8. Taste, and adjust seasoning accordingly.
9. Spread a generous amount of avocado pesto over each slice of toasted bread.
10. Serve and enjoy.

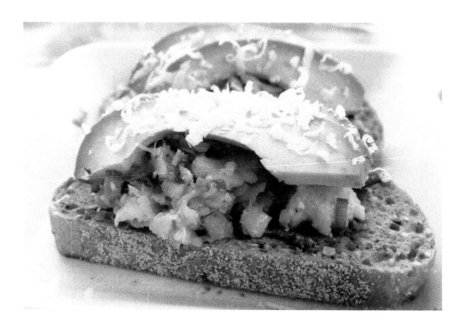

Sweet potatoes and black bean tostadas

This is a complete vegetarian Mediterranean recipe with roasted sweet potatoes serve beautifully on a bed of crisp salad.

Ingredients

- Salt
- Small handful of fresh cilantro leaves, chopped
- Extra virgin olive oil
- 1 teaspoon of ground cumin
- 2 cans of black beans, rinsed and drained
- Hot sauce or salsa
- ½ cup of water
- 2 cloves garlic, pressed
- 2 ripe avocados, pitted and thinly sliced
- ½ teaspoon sea salt grinder
- 8 corn of tortillas
- 18 ounces of romaine lettuce, roughly chopped
- 1 ¾ pounds of sweet potatoes
- ⅔ cup of feta cheese crumbles
- ½ teaspoon chili powder
- ¾ cup of finely chopped red onion, divided

- 2 tablespoons of fresh lime juice

Directions

1. Preheat the oven to 400°F.
2. Line baking sheets with parchment paper.
3. Place the sweet potatoes on baking sheets, drizzle with olive oil, and sprinkle with the chili powder and dash of salt. Toss to coat.
4. Let bake for 35 minutes, or until the sweet potatoes are tender and caramelized.
5. Warm olive oil over medium heat, until shimmering.
6. Then, add the garlic and cumin, let cook briefly, while stirring constantly.
7. Add drained beans, water and salt. Let simmer and cook for 10 minutes, stirring often.
8. Remove from the heat and mash the beans, cover and set aside.
9. On a baking sheet, brush both sides of each tortilla with oil.
10. Arrange 4 tortillas in a single layer across each pan.
11. Let bake for 12 minutes, turning until each tortilla is golden. Keep aside for later.
12. In a medium serving dish, combine the chopped lettuce together with the feta, red onion, olive oil, and lime juice. Toss to combine.

13. Divide the salad between 4 bowls.

14. Serve and enjoy immediately.

Kale, black bean, and avocado burrito bowl

Ingredients

- 3 cloves garlic, pressed
- ¼ teaspoon of salt
- 1 bunch of curly kale
- ¼ teaspoon of chili powder
- 2 tablespoons of olive oil
- ½ jalapeño, seeded and finely chopped
- ½ teaspoon of cumin
- Cherry tomatoes, sliced into thin rounds
- ¼ teaspoon of salt
- ¼ cup of lime juice
- 1 cup of brown rice, rinsed
- 1 avocado
- ½ cup of mild salsa Verde
- ¼ teaspoon of cayenne pepper
- ½ cup of fresh cilantro leaves
- Hot sauce
- 2 tablespoons of lime juice
- 2 cans of black beans, rinsed and drained
- 1 shallot, finely chopped

Directions

1. Bring a big pot of water to a boil, lace in the brown rice and boil, uncovered, for 30 minutes.

2. Drain any excess water, return to the pot. Let steam in the pot for 10 minutes, season with ¼ teaspoon salt and adjust accordingly.

3. Whisk the lime juice together with the olive oil, chopped jalapeño, cumin, and salt.

4. Toss the chopped kale with the lime marinade in a mixing bowl.

5. Combine the avocado chunks, salsa Verde, cilantro, and lime juice in a food processer, blend well.

6. Warm 1 tablespoon olive oil over medium-low heat.

7. Sauté the shallot together with the garlic until fragrant.

8. Add the beans with chili powder and cayenne pepper.

9. Let cook until the beans are warmed through in 7 minutes.

10. Serve and enjoy.

Sweet corn and black bean tacos

Beans are rich in protein; therefore, combining with variety of vegetables and fruits makes this recipe a perfect choice for Mediterranean Sea diet.

Ingredients

- 1 large avocado, sliced into thin strips
- Salt and black pepper
- 3 medium red radishes, thinly sliced into small strips
- ¼ cup of chopped cilantro
- 1 medium jalapeño pepper, seeded and minced
- 1 tablespoon of olive oil
- Pickled jalapeños, salsa Verde
- ¼ teaspoon of sea salt
- 2 ears of corn, shucked
- ⅔ cup of crumbled feta, to taste
- 1 medium lime, zested and juiced
- 2 cans of black beans, rinsed and drained
- 10 small round corn tortillas
- 1 tablespoon of olive oil
- 1 small yellow or white onion, chopped
- 1 tablespoon of ground cumin
- ⅓ cup of water

Directions

1. Place the kernels in a medium-sized mixing bowl with jalapeño, olive oil, chopped cilantro, radishes, lime zest and juice, and sea salt. Mix well.
2. Then, stir in crumbled feta, taste, and adjust.
3. Warm the olive oil over medium heat.
4. Add the onions with a sprinkle of salt, let cook 8 minutes, stirring occasionally.
5. Add the cumin, let cook briefly while stirring.
6. Pour in the beans and ⅓ cup water. Stir.
7. Lower the heat, let simmer, for 5 minutes, covered.
8. Smash half of the beans.
9. Remove from heat, then, season with salt and pepper.
10. Heat a cast iron over medium heat and warm each tortilla individually, flipping occasionally.
11. Serve and enjoy.

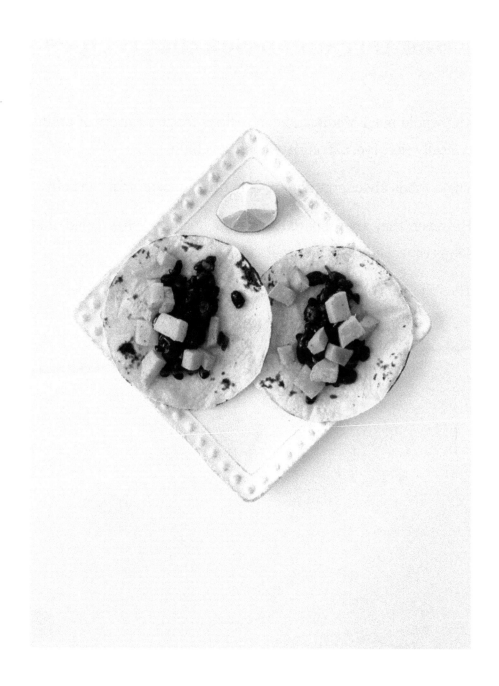

Whole meal and soup Mediterranean Sea diet recipes

The whole meal Mediterranean recipes feature variety of grains typically rice, rye, oat, corn, wheat, sorghum.

These foods are energy and carbohydrate boosters for the body.

However, they are prepared alongside healthy dishes, salad, and soups especially bean and seafood stew.

The following are the whole food Mediterranean Sea recipes.

Coconut millet bowl with berbere spiced squash and chickpeas

This is a plant based Mediterranean Sea diet that features shallots, spinach, millet grain, and coconut milk with vibrant flavors and spices.

Ingredients

- water
- 1 ½ lb. kabocha squash 3/4 slices
- 2 large shallots, sliced
- 1 cup of millet
- 1 teaspoon of grated fresh ginger
- 1 tablespoon of coconut oil
- ¼ cup of fresh mint leaves
- ¼ teaspoon of turmeric
- ¼ teaspoon salt
- ½ cup of fresh cilantro
- 15 oz. can chickpeas, drained
- 3 cups of fresh spinach
- ½ cup of coconut cream
- 2 tablespoons avocado oil

- ¼ cup of lime juice
- zest of one lime
- 1 teaspoon honey
- 2 tablespoons Berbere spice
- 1 cup of coconut milk
- ½ cup of cucumber chunks

Directions

1. Set your oven to 400°F.
2. Combine berbere , olive oil, and water in a bowl, hydrate for 10 minutes.
3. Set aside some coconut milk .
4. Boil the remaining coconut milk mixed with water, turmeric, and salt to a simmer.
5. Add coconut oil with millet bring to a gentle boil, lower heat, let simmer for 15 minutes covered.
6. Place prepared squash, shallots and chickpeas on sheet pan with parchment .
7. Spread the berbere paste with a brush.
8. Sprinkle with salt and place in oven for 30 minutes.
9. Combine and blend the reserved coconut cream, salt , honey , cucumber, lime juice, and zest, and fresh ginger until smooth.
10. Add the cilantro and mint, blend for few seconds.

11. Assemble the bowls with the veggies on top of the warm millet.
12. Then, add fresh spinach and drizzle with the sauce.
13. Serve and enjoy.

Pressure pot pinto bean stew

Ingredients

- 1 teaspoon of chipotle powder
- 2 teaspoons Molasses
- 1 tablespoon of olive oil
- 1 teaspoon of salt
- 1 large onion, chopped
- 4 cups of chopped poblano peppers
- 1 yam
- 4 cloves garlic coarsely chopped
- 14 oz. can of crushed tomatoes
- 3 cups of veggie broth
- 2 teaspoons of Ancho chili powder
- 1 cup of frozen corn
- 1 teaspoon of cumin
- 1 ½ cups of dry pinto beans
- 1 teaspoon of coriander

Directions

1. Set Pressure pot to Sauté.
2. Then, add olive oil with the onion, let sauté 5 minutes.
3. Add garlic and poblanos continue to sauté for 2 minutes.

4. Add the ancho chili powder together with the cumin, and coriander, stirring to coat.

5. Add the yams together with soaked beans, molasses, chipotle, tomatoes, chicken stock, and salt .

6. Set the Pressure Pot to high pressure for 25 minutes.

7. Manually release pressure valve.

8. Stir in frozen corn and let warm through.

9. Serve and enjoy.

Curried zucchini soup

Ingredients

- 2 teaspoons of yellow curry powder
- 2 tablespoons of coconut oil
- ¼ cup of cilantro- leaves
- 1 medium onion
- 2 cloves garlic
- 4 cups of chicken
- ¼ cup of mint leaves
- 1 tablespoon of ginger
- 1 jalapeño
- 1 ½ teaspoons of sea salt
- 2 pounds of zucchini or yellow squash

Directions

1. In a heavy-bottomed pot sauté onion with garlic, ginger, and jalapeño in coconut oil , for 5 minutes over medium heat.
2. Add the salt together with the zucchini and curry powder.
3. Sauté briefly.
4. Add 2 cups of the broth.

5. Let simmer, covered and cook until the summer squash is tender.
6. Add another 2 cups of cold broth to the a blender with all the simmered ingredients.
7. Blend, until smooth with a vented lid.
8. Add fresh mint and cilantro, blend to incorporated.
9. Serve and enjoy.

White bean chili with jackfruit

Ingredients

- 1 teaspoon of salt
- 1 tablespoon of coriander
- 1 tablespoon of cumin
- 2 tablespoons of olive oil
- 1 teaspoon of sugar
- 2 teaspoons of granulated garlic
- ½ teaspoon of pepper
- 1 onion, chopped
- 6 garlic cloves, rough chopped
- 2 teaspoons of dried oregano
- 1 poblano pepper, chopped
- 2 x 14-ounce cans of white beans
- ½ teaspoon of ground chipotle powder
- 16 ounces of canned jackfruit
- 3 cups of veggie broth
- 1 tablespoon of chili powder

Directions

1. Firstly, set your Pressure Pot to Sauté.
2. Then, heat 2 tablespoons of olive oil.

3. Add onion together with the garlic and fresh poblano, let sauté for 3 minutes until fragrant.
4. Add canned chilies together with the canned beans and jackfruit .
5. Add the veggie broth .
6. Add all the spice along with sugar and salt .
7. • Stir and set Pressure pot to a high heat for 10 minutes.
8. Naturally release the pressure.
9. Stir in corn with chopped kale and cover for 5 minutes on warm setting.
10. Taste, and adjust the seasoning.
11. Serve in bowls with diced avocado , cilantro, radishes.
12. Serve and enjoy.

Moroccan red lentil quinoa soup

Ingredients

- 2 tablespoons of olive oil
- 1 teaspoon of maple syrup
- 1 teaspoon of dried thyme
- 1 teaspoon of coriander
- 1 onion, diced
- 3/4 cup of red lentils
- 6 garlic cloves, rough chopped
- 3 carrots, diced
- 1 red bell pepper, diced
- 1 teaspoon of cinnamon
- ¼ cup of quinoa
- 1 poblano pepper, diced
- 1 14-ounce can of diced tomatoes
- 4 cups veggie broth
- 1 ½ teaspoon of salt
- 2 teaspoons of cumin
- 1 teaspoon of chili powder
- ½ teaspoon of turmeric

Directions

1. Set Pressure Pot to sauté function.

2. Heat olive oil.

3. Then, sauté the onion and garlic for 4 minutes, stirring until fragrant.

4. Add the carrots together with bell pepper, stir 2 minutes.

5. Add the diced tomatoes and broth.

6. Stir in the salt together with the cumin, chili powder, cinnamon, mable syrup, coriander, turmeric, and thyme .

7. • Stir in the split red lentils with the quinoa.

8. Set Pressure pot to high pressure for 5 minutes.

9. Manually release the pressure.

10. Taste, and adjust the seasoning.

11. Serve and enjoy with fresh radishes and herbs.

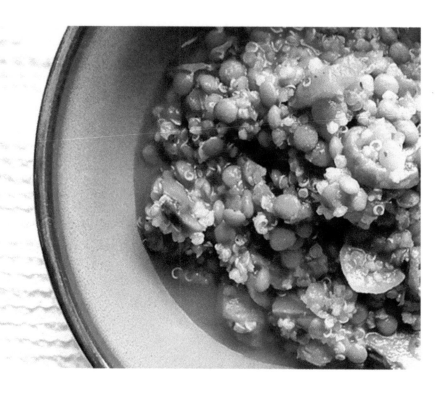

Potato wedges

Ingredients

- Olive oil
- Sea salt
- 600g of baking potatoes
- Freshly ground black pepper

Directions

1. Firstly, preheat your oven ready to 400°F.
2. Put a large pan of salted water to boil.
3. Add the potato wedges to the pan of boiling water let boil for 8 minutes.
4. Drain any excess water in a colander, let steam dry for briefly.
5. Transfer to a roasting tray.
6. Add olive oil together with a pinch of salt and pepper.
7. Toss to coat the wedges with oil, spread out in one layer.
8. Let cook in the hot oven for 30 minutes or until golden and cooked through.
9. Serve and enjoy with chicken or a dip.

Brothy tortellini soup with spinach, white beans, and basil

Ingredients

- 1 can of white beans
- 2 tablespoons of olive oil
- 8 ounces of chopped baby spinach
- 1 onion, diced
- 6 garlic cloves, rough chopped
- 1 teaspoon of salt
- 1 cup of fresh basil, chopped
- ½ teaspoon of pepper
- 1 cup of celery, diced
- 10 ounces of fresh tortellini
- 8 cups of veggie
- Squeeze of lemon
- 1 teaspoon of dry Italian herbs

Directions

1. Begin by heating olive oil in a large heavy bottom pot over medium-high heat.
2. Add the onion to sauté for 4 minutes, stirring.

3. Add the celery with garlic, lower heat to medium, let sauté for 6 minutes until celery is tender.

4. Add the broth, then raise the heat to high, bring to a boil.

5. Season with salt and Italian seasoning.

6. Add the fresh tortellini when boiling, let simmer for 5 minutes or until cooked.

7. Add the white beans and simmer briefly until heated through.

8. Add the chopped fresh spinach together with the basil, after turning off the heat.

9. Stir, and add a little squeeze of lemon.

10. Taste, and adjust the seasoning.

11. Serve and enjoy with a drizzle of olive oil , pecorino cheese and a light sprinkle of chili flakes.

Vegan ramen with shiitake broth

Ingredients

- 2 tablespoons of white miso paste
- 1 large onion-diced
- Pepper to taste
- 2 smashed garlic cloves
- Sriracha to taste
- 2 tablespoon of olive oil
- 8 ounces of Ramen Noodles
- 4 cups of veggie stock
- 8 ounces of cubed crispy tofu
- 4 cups of water
- ½ cup of dried Shiitake Mushrooms
- 1 sheet Kombu seaweed
- 1/8 cup of mirin

Directions

1. Sauté onion o ver medium-high heat in 1 tablespoon olive oil until tender about 3 minutes.
2. Turn heat to medium, add the smashed garlic cloves, let the onions cook until deeply golden brown.

3. Add the veggie stock with water, dried shiitakes, a sheet of kombu , and mirin . Let Simmer for 30 minutes uncovered.

4. R emove the Kombu .

5. Then, add the miso with pepper to taste.

6. In a pot of boiling water, cook the ramen noodles according to directions. Drain.

7. Toss with sesame oil to keep separated.

8. Sauté the spinach and mushrooms in olive oil until tender.

9. Seasoning with salt and pepper.

10. Fill bowls with cooked noodles, crispy tofu , and any other veggies.

11. Pour the flavorful Shiitake broth over top.

12. Serve and enjoy garnished with srirachi.

Cornbread casserole

Ingredients

- 2 large eggs
- 2 tablespoons of olive oil
- 1 cup of sour cream
- 1 onion, diced
- ¼ cup of melted butter
- 1 red bell pepper, diced
- 2 teaspoons of baking powder
- 4 cups of corn
- 1 ½ cups of grated cheese cheddar
- 4-ounce can of diced green chilies
- 1 teaspoon of cumin
- 1 teaspoon of coriander
- Salt
- 2 tablespoons chopped cilantro
- ½ cup of cornmeal
- 1 teaspoon of smoked paprika
- ½ cup of all-purpose flour
- 2 teaspoon of sugar

Directions

1. In a large skillet, over medium heat, sauté onion in olive oil until fragrant in 4 minutes.
2. Add the bell pepper, let cook for 4 minutes.
3. Add the fresh corn and let sauté for 4 minutes.
4. Stir in fresh cilantro.
5. In a large bowl, combine cornmeal together with the salt, flour, baking powder, and sugar, whisk.
6. In a separate medium bowl, whisk eggs with the sour cream. Then, gently whisk in the melted butter.
7. Add the sautéed corn/pepper mixture to the dry ingredients with the egg mixture, stir to combine.
8. Add 3/4 cup of grated cheese.
9. Pour the batter into the greased baking dish.
10. Topping with the remaining 3/4 cup of cheese.
11. Bake for 35 minutes uncovered.
12. Serve and enjoy warm sprinkled with cilantro.

Thai green curry

Ingredients

- Lime wedges for garnish
- ½ cup of homemade green curry paste
- 1 Japanese eggplant
- 1 teaspoon of sugar
- 2 tablespoons of olive oil
- 8 kefir lime leaves
- 1 cup of chicken broth
- ¼ cup of fresh Thai basil leaves, torn
- 1 can of coconut milk
- 8 ounces' pound of extra-firm tofu, cubed
- ½ teaspoon of salt
- 2 teaspoons of fish sauce
- 1 red bell pepper, sliced
- Lime juice to taste

Directions

1. Begin by heating olive oil in a heavy bottom pot over medium-high heat.
2. Stir-fry the homemade green curry paste for 3 minutes.
3. Add the stock, then Stir in one can of full coconut milk .
4. Add salt , sugar , and fish sauce

5. Add the tofu together with the veggies and kefir lime leaves.
6. Bring to a gentle simmer, uncovered until eggplant softens.
7. Add a squeeze of lime and taste, and adjust accordingly.
8. Add the fresh basil leaves and serve with lime wedges over rice.
9. Enjoy.

Kimchi burritos

Ingredients

- 1 cup of shredded cheese
- ½ cup of kimchi , chopped
- 2 tablespoon of olive oil
- 2 scallions, chopped
- 1 onion, diced
- Cilantro, hot sauce
- Salt to taste
- 1 red bell pepper, diced
- 1 cup of rice
- 1 can of black beans, rinsed, strained

Directions

1. In a large skillet, heat oil over medium heat.
2. Then, sauté onion with bell pepper for 5 minutes or until tender.
3. Add rice together with kimchi and black beans, stir to combine.
4. Season with salt and scallions.
5. Taste, and adjust spices accordingly.
6. Add cheese to the pan, gently melt, stirring for until melty and stringy.

7. Divide filling into the center of the warm tortillas.

8. Top with hot sauce and or cilantro and wrap into a burrito.

9. Serve and enjoy immediately.

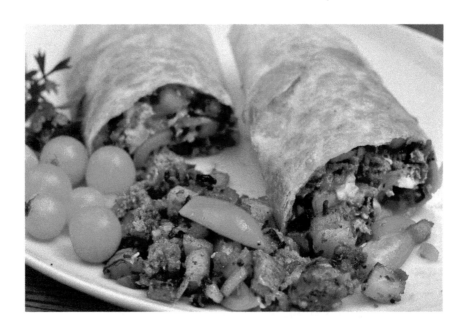

Singapore style fried rice

This specific Mediterranean Sea diet recipe has many variations with a perfect seasoning and fluffiness, if can be blended with various vegetables of your liking.

Ingredients

- 1 teaspoon of chili jam
- 4 fresh or frozen raw peeled prawns
- 150g of brown
- 1 teaspoon of mixed seeds
- 320g of crunchy veggies
- 1 tablespoon of low-salt soy sauce
- 1 teaspoon of tikka paste
- 1 rasher of smoked streaky bacon
- 1 clove of garlic
- 2cm of piece of ginger
- 1 large free-range egg
- Olive oil
- 1 chipolata

Directions

1. Start by cooking the rice according as per packet Directions.
2. Drain any excess water let cool.
3. Put a large non-stick frying pan on a medium-high heat.
4. Place 1 teaspoon of olive oil into the hot pan.
5. Pour in the egg, swirl around the pan.
6. Cook through, remove and roll up and slice.
7. Put ½ a tablespoon of olive oil into the hot pan.
8. Stir-fry the bacon with sausages until golden.
9. Add the prawns with garlic and ginger.
10. Stir in the curry paste to coated everything.
11. Add the vegetables, begin with hard to cook veggies. Keep stirring.
12. Place in the cool rice and stir-fry until the veggies are just cooked.
13. Add the soy, toss in the egg ribbons.
14. Divide between plates, sprinkle over the seeds.
15. Season and adjust accordingly.
16. Serve and enjoy with a drizzle of chili jam.

Purple cauliflower salad

Ingredients

- 2 tablespoons of red wine vinegar
- ½ cup of Italian parsley, chopped
- 1 head cauliflower
- ½ teaspoon of pepper
- 2 cloves garlic, minced
- Salt
- zest of one lemon
- 2 cups of cooked grain- black rice
- 2 scallions, sliced
- ½ cup of sliced Kalamata olives
- 2 tablespoons of capers
- olive oil

Directions

1. Preheat your oven to 425°F.
2. Set grains to cook on the stove.
3. Remove and let cool.
4. Cut cauliflower into bite-sized florets.
5. Then, slightly toss in olive oil , salt and lemon zest.
6. Spread out on a parchment -lined baking sheet.

7. Let roast for 25 minutes, turning halfway through. Let cool.
8. In a bowl, whisk olive oil, red wine vinegar, garlic, salt, and pepper.
9. Layer salad ingredients in a shallow bowl starting with the grain.
10. Serve and enjoy.

Grilled cabbage with andouille sausage

Ingredients

- 1 tablespoon of olive oil
- 1 tablespoon of fresh chives
- 2 tablespoons of whole grain mustard
- 1 ½ tablespoons of honey
- 1 large purple cabbage
- Olive oil for brushing
- Salt and pepper
- 6 andouille sausages
- ¼ teaspoon of salt
- ¼ teaspoon of pepper
- 2 tablespoons of apple cider vinegar

Directions

1. Preheat your grill on high heat.
2. Grease the grill well.
3. Brush each side of cabbage with olive oil .
4. Season with salt and pepper.
5. lower grill to medium heat, then add sausages and thinly sliced cabbage.

6. Grill the cabbage for 8 minutes on both sides.

7. Grill the sausages until seared.

8. Place cabbage steaks down on a large platter.

9. Spoon half of the dressing over top.

10. Slice the sausages in half and steep diagonal and scatter over cabbage.

11. Serve and enjoy garnished with chopped chives.

Superfood walnut pesto noodles

Ingredients

- ¼ cup of sliced radishes
- 1 cup of walnuts
- ¼ cup of walnuts
- 2 tablespoons of sesame oil
- 4 ounces of dry soba noodles
- 1 cup of power greens
- Squeeze of lemon to taste
- 2 tablespoons of white miso
- Olive oil and lemon for drizzling
- 2 garlic cloves, start with one
- ¼ cup water
- 4 cups of baby superfood greens
- ½ cup of shredded cabbage
- Edamame, sunflower sprouts, avocado , snow peas

Directions

1. Cook soba noodles according to the package ins
2. Place walnuts together with the miso , olive oil, garlic, and water into a food processor, blend repeatedly.
3. Then, add the power greens and pulse.
4. Taste and adjust the taste and consistence.

5. Toss the noodles with walnut pesto.
6. Place noodles in a bento box with a handful of greens, shredded cabbage, walnuts, and radishes.
7. Drizzle vegetables with a little olive oil , lemon, and salt .
8. Serve and enjoy.

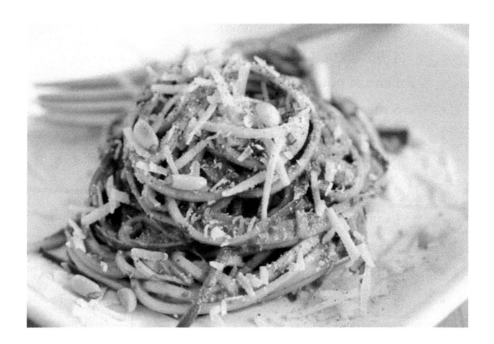

Carrots soup with chermoula

Ingredients

- ½ a large onion
- 1 tablespoon of lemon juice
- 1 ½ teaspoon of Cumin seeds
- ¼ teaspoon of salt
- 4 garlic cloves, smashed
- 4 cups chicken stock
- 2 bay leaves
- Zest from ½ lemon
- 1 teaspoon of kosher salt
- ¼ teaspoon of white pepper
- ¼ teaspoon of chili flakes
- 2 teaspoons of honey
- ¼ cup of yogurt
- 1 teaspoon of cumin seeds , toasted
- 1 lbs. carrots, cut into disks
- 1 teaspoon of fresh thyme
- 1 teaspoon coriander seeds, toasted
- 1 cup of cilantro
- ½ cup of Italian parsley
- 1 teaspoon of fresh ginger
- 2 garlic cloves
- Olive oil

Directions

1. Sauté onion together with the cumin seeds and smashed garlic in olive oil over medium high heat until golden, stirring often.
2. Add carrots with chicken stock, bay leaves, salt , white pepper .
3. Bring to a vigorous simmer, lower, simmer covered for 20 minutes over low heat.
4. Then, toast the spices in a dry skillet over medium heat until fragrant.
5. Combine all ingredients in a food processor , blend to form paste. Keep aside for later.
6. Blend the soup using an immersion blender or in small batches.
7. Place back in the pot, stir in sour cream and maple syrup .
8. Taste, and adjust seasoning.
9. Divide among bowls, then add a spoonful of chermoula, swirl in a circle.
10. Serve and enjoy.

Lemony corona beans with olive and garlic

Ingredients

- Salt and pepper to taste
- 2 teaspoons of kosher salt
- ¼ cup of fresh parsley leaves
- 2 bay leaves
- 3 celery sticks, cut into pieces
- Aleppo chili flakes
- 1 onion, quartered
- zest of one lemon
- 1 lb. dry Royal Corona Beans
- 4 garlic cloves, smashed
- A few fresh sage leaves
- 3 tablespoons of olive oil

Directions

1. Place soaked beans in a large Dutch oven with water enough to cover them.
2. Add salt together with the celery, garlic, onion, bay leaves, and herbs.

3. Bring to a boil, lower heat, let simmer covered until tender n about 2 hours.

4. Drain, reserve some liquid without the aromatics for later.

5. Place in a serving dish .

6. Then, add back 1 cup of the reserved warm cooking liquid with olive oil , lemon zest, fresh Italian parsley, and salt and pepper.

7. Serve and enjoy.

Szechuan tofu and vegetables

Ingredients

- 1 cup of asparagus, snap peas
- 12 ounces of tofu, patted dry, cubed
- ¼ cup of Szechuan Sauce
- 1 cup of shredded carrots
- 2 tablespoons of peanut oil
- generous pinch of salt and pepper
- ½ red bell pepper, thinly sliced
- ½ cup of thinly sliced onion
- Scallions of sesame seeds
- 4 ounces of sliced mushrooms
- 2 cups of shredded cabbage

Directions

1. Heat olive oil in a skillet over medium heat.
2. Season peanut oil together with salt and pepper.
3. Then, swirl the seasoned peanut oil to spread out uniformly.
4. Add tofu and sear on at least two sides, until crispy and golden.
5. In the same pan, add onion and mushrooms.

6. Sauté over medium-high heat, stirring constantly, until tender.
7. Add the remaining vegetables with dried red chilies
8. Lower heat to medium, sauté, while tossing and stirring for 5 minutes.
9. Add the Szechuan Sauce , gradually.
10. Let cook for 2 minutes, until thickened a bit.
11. Toss in the crispy tofu towards the end.
12. Divide among bowls.
13. Sprinkle with sesame seeds and scallions.
14. Serve and enjoy with noodles or over rice.

Kyoto roasted sweet potatoes with miso, ginger, and scallions

Ingredients

- Salt to taste
- 3 yams sliced in half
- 2 teaspoons of ginger finely minced
- 3 Scallions, sliced
- Olive oil for brushing
- 1 tablespoon of miso
- ¼ cup of olive oil
- 1 large shallot, finely diced

Directions

1. Preheat your oven ready to 425°F.
2. Place cut sweet potatoes on a parchment -lined sheet pan
3. Brush with olive oil .
4. Let roast for 40 minutes until fork tender.
5. Heat the olive oil over medium low heat.
6. Then, add the shallot to sauté until golden, stirring often.
7. Add the ginger, continue to cook for 3 more minutes.
8. Add and mash the miso with a fork into the mixture. Turn off the heat.

9. After the sweet potatoes are caramelized, remove and place on a platter flesh side up.
10. Reheat the miso, pierce the flesh in a few spots, spoon a tablespoon of the sauce over each one with the flavor.
11. Sprinkle with a little finishing salt and scallions.
12. Serve and enjoy.

Wonton soup

Ingredients

- Chopped greens
- 1 leek, white parts, thinly sliced
- Scallions, cilantro, sesame seeds
- 4 slices ginger
- Salt and lemon juice to taste
- 1 tablespoon of olive oil
- 4 cups of chicken broth
- 14 wontons

Directions

1. In a medium pot , sauté the shallot with ginger in olive oil, over medium heat, until fragrant.
2. Add the broth, cover and bring to a boil.
3. Add the wontons and simmer according to directions on the package.
4. Taste, and adjust the seasoning accordingly.
5. Place in the greens let cook until wilted.
6. Spinach and kale take more time compared to others.
7. Divide between two bowls, then sprinkle with cilantro, scallions, and sesame seeds.
8. Enjoy.

Roasted Portobello steaks with walnut coffee sauce

Ingredients

- 1 teaspoon of miso
- 4 garlic cloves, chopped
- 4 extra-large Portobello mushrooms
- 5 tablespoons of olive oil
- ½ teaspoon of pepper
- ½ teaspoon of salt
- 1 teaspoon of balsamic
- Generous pinch salt and pepper
- 2 extra-large shallots, rough diced
- 1 cup of walnuts, raw
- 1 tablespoon of balsamic vinegar
- 1 ¼ cup of black coffee
- Drizzle of truffle oil , a spring of thyme

Directions

1. Preheat oven ready to 400°F.
2. Then, mix olive oil together with the vinegar in a small bowl.
3. Use it to brush the Portobello on both sides.

4. Season, or sprinkle with salt and pepper and place gills side down, on a parchment lined sheet pan .

5. Let bake until tender in 25 minutes.

6. Wrap in foil until ready to use.

7. Heat another olive oil in a medium sauce pan, over medium heat.

8. Sauté the shallots with the garlic until fragrant and tender, stirring often.

9. Add the walnuts and stir for 2 minutes.

10. Add the coffee, scraping up any brown bits.

11. Pour into a blender with salt , pepper, miso paste, balsamic.

12. Then, blend until silky smooth.

13. Place the sauce back in the pan and heat up gently before plating.

14. When the Portobello are done, slice and place over the Coffee Walnut sauce in a serving dish .

15. Top with a sprig of thyme and pomegranate seeds .

16. Serve and enjoy.

Vegan tomato soup with coconut, ginger, and turmeric

Ingredients

- 3/4 teaspoon of salt
- 2 tablespoons of olive oil
- 1 14 ounce can of coconut milk
- 2 fat shallots, rough chopped
- 3 garlic cloves, rough chopped
- Peanut Chili Crunch and Scallions
- 1 tablespoon of ginger, rough chopped
- 1 14 ounces can of diced tomatoes
- 2 teaspoons of fresh turmeric, rough chopped
- 1 cup of water
- ¼ teaspoon of cayenne
- 1 tablespoon of tomato paste

Directions

1. Begin by Sautéing the shallot together with the garlic, ginger, and fresh turmeric in a medium pot , over medium heat in olive oil, until deeply golden.
2. Add the tomato paste, stir for 1 minute.

3. Transfer to a blender with the can of tomatoes, puree until so smooth.

4. Return back to the same pot.

5. Add 1 cup of water with can of coconut milk , ground turmeric, salt , and cayenne.

6. Bring to a simmer, turn off heat, taste, and adjust the seasoning accordingly.

7. Divide among bowls and top with Peanut Chili Crunch and scallions.

8. Serve and enjoy.

Roasted parsnips with romesco sauce

Ingredients

- 1 teaspoon of cumin
- 3 extra-large parsnips
- ½ teaspoon of chili flakes
- ¾ teaspoon of salt
- 1 red bell pepper, halved
- 1 tablespoon of tomato paste
- ¾ inch thick wedges of onions
- 1 tablespoon of sherry wine vinegar
- Salt and pepper
- 1 teaspoon of smoked paprika
- ¼ cup of chopped fresh Italian parsley
- 2 garlic cloves
- Olive oil
- ¼ cup of water
- ½ cup of toasted hazelnuts

Directions

1. Preheat oven to 425°F.

2. Place parsnips and bell pepper on a parchment lined sheet pan .

3. Add onion wedges to the pan.

4. Brush with olive oil all over.

5. Season and or sprinkle with salt and pepper.

6. Let roast for 35 minutes until fork tender.

7. Place bell pepper and onion in a food processor .

8. Add remaining romesco ingredients and pulse to form paste.

9. The, spoon the romesco sauce onto a platter, smear all over.

10. Arrange the parsnips overtop.

11. Sprinkle with chopped parsley and crushed hazelnuts .

12. Serve and enjoy immediately.

Szechuan chicken and Brussels sprouts

Ingredients

- 1 tablespoon fresh ginger
- 2 lbs. chicken thighs
- 1 teaspoon salt , more for sprinkling
- 1 ½ lbs. medium Brussel sprouts, halved
- 1 tablespoon of sesame oil
- 4 fat garlic cloves, finely minced
- 1 teaspoon of Szechuan peppercorns
- ¼ cup of honey
- ¼ cup of soy sauce
- 1 tablespoon of rice vinegar
- Scallions
- 3 teaspoons of garlic chili paste

Directions

1. Preheat oven to 425°F.
2. Combine honey, soy sauce, rice vinegar, sesame oil, chili paste, garlic, ginger, salt, and Szechuan peppercorns in a medium bowl.
3. Pour half of the marinade over the chicken.

4. Place and lock in a bag, let marinate.

5. Place Brussel sprouts in a bowl, then pour the remaining marinade over Brussel sprouts, toss.

6. Nestle the chicken thighs in between, and spoon any remaining marinade over the chicken.

7. Season the chicken with a little salt.

8. Let b ake for 30 minutes in the preheated oven, checking at 20 minutes.

9. Divide the Brussel sprouts and top with the chicken.

10. Sprinkle with scallions.

11. Serve and enjoy.

Palak paneer

Ingredients

- ¾ cup of plain yogurt
- 1 paneer
- ½ cup of cashews
- 1 cup of water
- 12 ounces of frozen spinach
- 3 tablespoons of ghee
- Squeeze lemon
- 1 teaspoon of salt
- 1 white onion, diced
- 2 tablespoons of ginger, rough chopped
- ½ teaspoon of sugar
- 4 garlic cloves, rough chopped
- 1 jalapeno
- 2 teaspoons of cumin
- 2 teaspoons of coriander
- 2 teaspoons of Garam masala
- 1 teaspoon of black mustard seeds

Directions

1. In a large skillet, heat bit of ghee.
2. Season the ghee with salt and pepper.

3. Then, pan-sear the paneer until golden and crispy.

4. Wipe out the skillet, heat 3 tablespoons of ghee over medium heat.

5. Add onion together with the ginger, garlic, and chilies.

6. Sauté for 15 minutes, or until deeply golden and fragrant, stirring often.

7. Add coriander together with the cumin , Garam masala , and mustard seeds, let sauté 3 more minutes.

8. Add the frozen spinach and cup of water, over low heat, simmer uncovered until the spinach is thawed.

9. Transfer to a blender , top with the yogurt and cashews.

10. Add the salt and sugar , then, blend until silky smooth.

11. If salty, add the paneer to soak the salt.

12. Place the blended spinach sauce back into the pan uncovered, on med-low heat.

13. Add the pan-seared paneer and continue cooking until the paneer is warmed through.

14. Serve and enjoy over naan Bread or cauliflower rice .

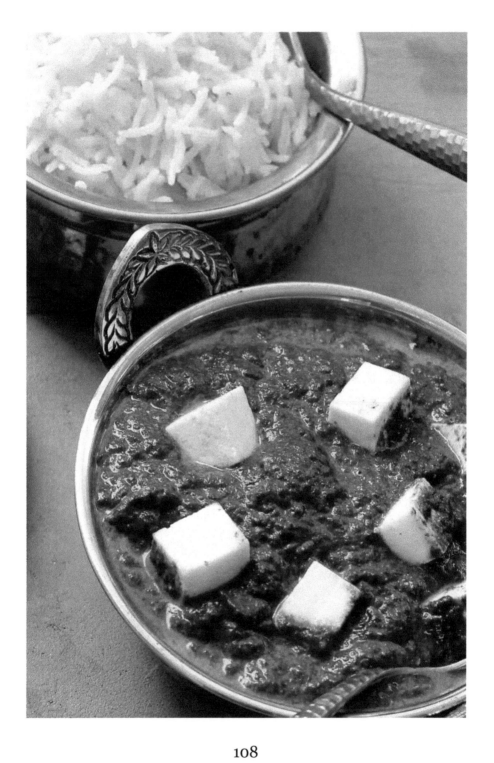

Lightning Source UK Ltd.
Milton Keynes UK
UKHW020843040621
384920UK00001B/40